Autoimmune Retinopathy (AIR)

Frances Foster, MS, NP
Ryon Yu
Zihan Yu
C. Stephen Foster, MD, FACS, FACR

To all our patients with AutoImmune Retinopathy
...and to the quest for a cure

Autoimmune Retinopathy (AIR)

ISBN: 978-1-7332376-8-0

The Ocular Immunology and Uveitis Foundation is a 501c(3), not-for-profit, tax-exempt organization. Our mission is to find cures for ocular inflammatory diseases, to correct the world-wide deficit of properly trained ocular immunologists, and to provide education and emotional support for those patients afflicted with ocular inflammatory disease.

OIUF

THE OCULAR IMMUNOLOGY AND UVEITIS FOUNDATION

Dedicated to Eye Disease Cure and Education

Eye words to know

Retina: Layer of nerve cells lining the back wall inside the eye. This layer senses light and sends signals to the brain so you can see.

Autoimmune: An autoimmune disease is a condition in which your immune system mistakenly attacks your body and releases proteins called autoantibodies to attack healthy cells.

Retinopathy: Retinopathy is any damage to the retina of the eyes, which may cause vision impairment. Retinopathy often refers to retinal vascular disease, damage to the retina caused by abnormal blood flow.

Paraneoplastic: A paraneoplastic disease is a disease associated with the presence of a cancerous growth, also called a *neoplasm*, in the body. The presence of the cancer can cause an overactive autoimmune response to target healthy cells in the eye.

What is autoimmune Retinopathy (AIR)?

Autoimmune retinopathy (AIR) is an immune disorder in which auto-antibodies produced by the immune system attack the retina, the nerve, or both, leading to progressive vision loss.

There are two forms of AIR: paraneoplastic and nonparaneoplastic retinopathy.

• **Paraneoplastic retinopathy *(pAIR)*** pAIR is divided into two sub-categories.

- **Cancer-associated retinopathy *(CAR)***
- **Melanoma-associated retinopathy *(MAR)***

• **Nonparaneoplastic retinopathy *(npAIR)*** npAIR is not associated with cancer and more likely occurs in patients with autoimmune disease.

- Nonparaneoplastic retinopathy is the more common form of AIR.

What causes AIR?

The immune system naturally produces anti- bodies to target pathogens and cancerous cells. However, mistakenly produced antibodies may target healthy retinal cells causing retinopathy (antibodies targeting the optic nerve can cause *neuropathy*). There are certain auto-antibodies known to contribute to AIR, and these can be tested for in serologic testing.

In some patients, the cause can be linked to retinal inflammation, hereditary retinal degeneration, or a history of autoimmune disease.

What are symptoms of AIR?

You can have AIR without knowing it. AIR can cause sudden, progressive and painless vision loss. As it worsens, you may notice symptoms such as:

- Seeing flashes of light
- Trouble dealing with bright light and/or dim light
- Decreased color vision
- Dark areas in your field of vision
- Poor night vision

Symptoms of autoimmune retinopathy usually affect both eyes but not always to the same extent.

How is AIR diagnosed?

- During an eye exam, your ophthalmologist will observe clinical signs.
- Diagnosis of AIR is made based on a careful review of history and clinical examination.

The examination may include the following:

-**Serologic testing** is a blood test used to detect the antibodies that are circulating in the blood serum, which may be attacking the retina. This test is performed in the same way as a standard blood test.

-**Optical coherence tomography *(OCT)*** is a way to look closely at the retina. A machine scans the retina and provides detailed images of its thickness. This helps your doctor examine the health of your retinal layers.

-**Fluorescein angiography** is a test in which a yellow dye (called fluorescein) is injected into a vein, usually in your arm. The dye travels through your blood vessels. A special camera takes photos of the retina as the dye travels throughout its blood vessels. This reveals blood vessels that are blocked or leaking fluid.

-**Full-field electroretinography** ***(ffERG)*** is a diagnostic test that can measure the responsiveness of retinal cells to light stimulus. This test can determine the type of cells that is being targeted and how the loss of those cells causes vision loss.

- **Cancer screening** may be recommended. Symptoms of AIR can onset after or even before a systemic diagnosis for cancer. Therefore, it is pertinent to conduct a thorough review for cancer to determine the proper treatment.

How is AIR treated?

Your treatment follows a step ladder approach and will be based on your ophthalmologist's diagnosis of your condition and cause. In patients with CAR, treating the cancer systemically often treats the retinopathy as well. Because AIR is associated with dysfunction of the immune system, ***immuno-suppression therapy*** is the most effective treatment to stabilize your condition and to potentially recover lost vision.

Immunosuppression therapy attempts to re-program the immune system to prevent attack of the body's own cells and to put the disease in remission. In our experience, the most ideal or effective therapy is intravenous Rituximab plus/minus Intravenous Immunoglobin G and Velcade subcutaneous injection.

Stepladder Approach for Immunosuppression Therapy

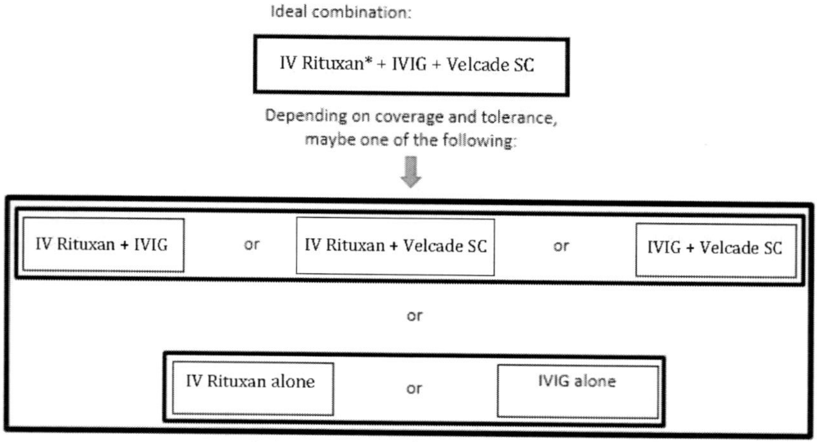

* Rituxan is the preferred brand of Rituximab
IV= Intravenous / SC = Subcutaneous Injection

Drug side effects:

Rituxan: Most Common: Fatigue, Headache, dyspepsia, fever, chills, joint or muscle aches, nausea, lower your body's ability to fight infection or cause allergic reaction. Tell your health care provider if you develop any signs of infection such as fever, chills, cough, sore throat, etc. To lower your risk of adverse effects, your doctor may add premedications and tell you to drink plenty of fluids before infusion

IVIG: Most people handle IVIG well, but most common side effects can include low-grade fever, muscle or joint aches, fatigue, and headaches just after your infusion. You might feel your best soon after your treatment, when the highest amount of immunoglobulin is in your body. To lower your risk of adverse effects, your doctor may add a pre- medication before infusion and tell you to drink plenty of fluids.

Velcade: Most Common: Fatigue, headache, joint or muscle aches, or pain and redness at injection site. Velcade can lower your body's ability to fight an infection. Tell your doctor if you develop signs of an infection such as fever, chills, or persistent sore throat.

With any medication, watch for signs of allergic reaction such as body rash/hives, itchy throat, swelling of lips, or other signs of anaphylaxis. Call for emergency medical care if any occur.

References:

1. Adamus G, Ren G, Weleber RG. Autoantibodies against retinal proteins in paraneoplastic and auto-immune retinopathy. *BMC Ophthalmology.* 2004;4(1)

2. Autoimmune Retinopathy. Oregon Health & Science University. https://www.ohsu.edu/xd/health/services/casey-eye/clinical-services/specialty-services/genetics/autoimmune-retinopathy.cfm. Accessed June 25, 2019.

3. Berge JCT, Rosmalen JV, Vermeer J, et al. Serum Autoantibody Profiling of Patients with Paraneoplastic and Non-Paraneoplastic Autoimmune Retinopathy. *Plos One.* 2016;11(12)

4. Canamary AM, Takahashi WY, Sallum JMF. Auto- immune retinopathy: A Review. *International Journal of Retina and Vitreous.* 2018;4(1)

5. Dy I, Chintapatla R, Preeshagul I, Becker D. Treatment of Cancer-Associated Retinopathy With Rituximab. *Journal of the National Comprehensive Cancer Network.* 2013;11(11):1320-1324

6. Khanna S, Ringeisen A, Mititelu M. Diagnosis and Management of Autoimmune Retinopathy. American Academy of Ophthalmology. https://www.aao.org/eyenet/article/diagnosis-and-management-of-autoimmune-retinopathy.Published October 16, 2017. Accessed June 25, 2019.

7. Silverman GJ, Weisman S. Rituximab therapy and autoimmune disorders: Prospects for anti-B cell therapy. *Arthritis & Rheumatism*. 2003;48(6): 1484-1492

8. Uludag G, Onal S, Arf S, et al. Electroretinographic improvement after rituximab therapy in a patient with autoimmune retinopathy. *American Journal of Ophthalmology* Case Reports. 2016;2:4-7

The Ocular Immunology and Uveitis Foundation is a 501c(3), not-for-profit, tax-exempt organization. Our mission is to find cures for ocular inflammatory diseases, to correct the worldwide deficit of properly trained ocular immunologists, and to provide education and emotional support for those patients afflicted with ocular inflammatory disease.

We Believe…

- In this day and age, no patients should suffer with poor treatment for ocular inflammatory disease.
- A cure is possible for ocular inflammatory disease.
- We can correct the deficit of properly trained ocular immunologists.
- Patients should have ample support during this time of need.

www.uveitis.org

OIUF

THE OCULAR IMMUNOLOGY AND UVEITIS FOUNDATION

Dedicated to Eye Disease Cure and Education

Notes

Made in United States
North Haven, CT
04 November 2026

21765611R00015